~~Eradicating~~ *LIVER* Diseases

The ultimate guide to putting an end to Hepatitis, Cirrhosis, Hemochromatosis, NAFLD, Liver Cancer, Cholangitis among others

Dr. Madelyn Reyes

Table of Contents

Chapter One
Introduction

Any illness that directly affects the liver is considered a liver ailment. Acute liver failure occurs quickly, whereas liver disease advances gradually over time.

The liver performs a variety of vital tasks, including as breaking down and transporting nutrients in food.

Liver illnesses and ailments come in a variety of forms. Some are brought on by viruses, such as hepatitis. Others may be brought on by drug use or excessive alcohol consumption. Cirrhosis can be brought on by a persistent injury or scar tissue in the liver. One indicator of liver disease is jaundice, or yellowing of the skin.

A healthy adult liver is around the size of a football. It is located directly beneath your rib cage on the right side of your abdomen. Your doctor may feel your liver by pressing on your abdomen if it's enlarged, or larger than it should be.

Frequency of Liver Diseases

In the US, liver illness is widespread. More than 100 million adults truly suffer from liver disease, despite the fact that only 4.5 million adults (1.8%) are officially diagnosed with it. They simply are ignorant.

With over 55,000 fatalities annually, liver disease ranks as the ninth most prevalent cause of mortality in the United States. Certain racial and ethnic groups are also more affected by the disease than others. For instance, compared to non-Hispanic White men, Black men have a 60% higher risk of developing liver-related cancers and passing away from them. In comparison to non-Hispanic White women, Black women also die from liver-related cancer at a higher rate (30% more likely).

Liver illness comes in several forms. Some are inherited (you are born with them), while others are brought on by viruses, diseases, or poisons like alcohol or drugs. The following list includes a few liver-related illnesses:

Alcoholic Hepatitis

Alcohol consumption causes inflammation, or swelling, of the liver, which is known as alcoholic hepatitis. Alcohol use damages liver tissue.

The majority of cases of alcoholic hepatitis occur in heavy drinkers over long periods of time. However, there is more to alcoholic hepatitis than meets the eye. Alcoholic hepatitis does not always strike big drinkers. And individuals who use even less alcohol develop the illness.

You have to give up alcohol consumption if you are diagnosed with alcoholic hepatitis. Alcohol abusers are at a higher risk of fatalities and severe liver damage.

Symptoms

Jaundice, or the yellowing of the skin and eye whites, is the most typical symptom of alcoholic hepatitis. People of color, such as Blacks and Browns, may have less noticeable skin yellowing.

Additional signs and symptoms consist of:

- Loss of appetite
- Nausea and vomiting
- discomfort in the belly
- fever, frequently of mild grade
- Weakness and fatigue

Alcoholic hepatitis patients frequently have low blood sugar. People who consume huge amounts of alcohol do not experience hunger. And alcohol is where heavy drinkers receive the majority of their calories.

Additional signs and symptoms of severe alcohol-related hepatitis include:

- Ascites is an accumulation of fluid in the abdomen.

- being poisoned to the point of confusion and abnormal behavior. These pollutants are broken down and eliminated by a healthy liver.
- liver and kidney damage.

When to see a doctor

Alcoholic hepatitis is a dangerous illness that can be fatal.

Consult a medical expert if you:

- possess alcoholic hepatitis symptoms.
- unable to limit your alcohol intake.
- Wish to reduce the amount of alcohol you consume

Causes

Alcohol consumption damages the liver, which results in alcoholic hepatitis. It's unclear exactly how alcohol harms the liver and why it only affects certain heavy drinkers.

Alcoholic hepatitis is known to be influenced by the following factors:

- Alcohol is broken down by the body into extremely harmful substances.

- These substances cause inflammation, or swelling, which kills liver cells.
- Healthy liver tissue eventually gives way to scarring. As a result, the liver cannot function properly.
- There is no cure for this scarring, known as cirrhosis. It's the final stage of alcoholic liver disease.

Additional variables associated with alcohol-related hepatitis include:

- **Other types of liver disease:** Steroid-induced hepatitis can exacerbate long-term liver damage. For example, there is a higher risk of liver damage if you have hepatitis C and drink, even in moderation.
- **Lack of nutrition:** Many heavy drinkers eat badly, which prevents them from getting enough nutrients in their diet. Additionally, alcohol prevents the body from properly utilizing nutrients. Nutrient deficiencies can harm hepatic cells.

Risk factors

The amount of alcohol you drink is the main risk factor for developing alcoholic hepatitis. The amount of alcohol required to cause alcoholic hepatitis is unknown.

Most patients with this illness have consumed seven or more drinks per day for at least 20 years. This could be seven shots of liquor, seven beers, or seven glasses of wine.

But even those with lower alcohol consumption may develop alcoholic hepatitis if they have additional risk factors, such as:

- **Sex:** It appears that women are more likely to get alcoholic hepatitis. That could be due to the way women's bodies metabolize alcohol.

- **Obesity:** Overweight heavy drinkers may be at higher risk of developing alcoholic hepatitis and ultimately developing liver scarring.

- **Genes:** Studies indicate that alcohol-induced liver damage may be influenced by genes.

- **Race and ethnicity:** There may be an increased risk of alcoholic hepatitis among Black and Hispanic individuals.

- **Binge drinking:** Alcohol-related hepatitis may become more likely in men who consume five or more drinks in a two-hour period, and in women who consume four or more.

Complications

Liver scar tissue is the cause of complications associated with alcohol-induced hepatitis. Hepatic blood flow can be slowed by scar tissue. Toxin accumulation may result from this increase in pressure in the portal vein, a significant blood artery.

Among the complications are:

Enlarged veins, called varices: When the portal vein is restricted, blood can back up into other stomach blood vessels and the esophagus, the tube that transports food from the throat to the stomach.

The walls of these blood arteries are thin. If they are overfilled with blood, they will probably bleed. Severe bleeding in the esophagus or upper stomach is life-threatening and requires immediate medical attention.

- **Ascites:** Stomach fluid accumulation may get infected and require antibiotic treatment. There is no risk to life from ascites. However, it typically indicates cirrhosis or severe alcoholic hepatitis.

- **Confusion, drowsiness and slurred speech, called hepatic encephalopathy:** Toxins are difficult for a damaged liver to eliminate from the body. Toxin accumulation can cause harm to the brain. Coma may result from severe hepatic encephalopathy.

- **Kidney failure:** Liver disease might impact the kidneys' blood supply. The kidneys may suffer from this.

- **Cirrhosis:** Liver failure may result from this liver scarring.

Liver Cancer

Cancer that starts in the cells of your liver is known as liver cancer. Located in the top right section of your abdomen, beneath your diaphragm and above your stomach, lies your liver, an organ the size of a football.

The liver can develop into several forms of cancer. Hepatocellular carcinoma is the most prevalent kind of liver cancer, and it starts in the primary hepatocyte form of liver cell. Hepatoblastoma and intrahepatic cholangiocarcinoma are two less prevalent forms of liver cancer.

Compared to cancer that starts in the liver cells, cancer that spreads to the liver occurs more frequently. Metastatic cancer, as opposed to liver cancer, is the term for cancer that starts in another part of the body, such as the colon, lung, or breast, and then spreads to the liver. This kind of cancer is called after the organ in which it first appeared; for example, cancer that starts in the colon and travels to the liver is called metastatic colon cancer.

Symptoms

In the early stages of primary liver cancer, the majority of people don't exhibit any symptoms or indicators. When symptoms do materialize, they could include the following:

- Getting in shape without making an effort
- appetite decline
- ache in the upper abdomen
- vomiting and nausea
- overall weakness and exhaustion
- stomach edema
- Jaundice is the yellow staining of the whites of your eyes and skin.
- Chalky white stools

When to see a doctor

Schedule a visit with your physician if you see any warning signs or symptoms that concern you.

Causes

When liver cells experience DNA alterations, or mutations, liver cancer results. The molecule that gives instructions for each and every chemical reaction in your body is called DNA.

These instructions vary as a result of DNA mutations. One outcome could be the start of uncontrollably growing cells that eventually develop into a tumor, which is a mass of malignant cells.

Sometimes, as in the case of persistent hepatitis infections, the cause of liver cancer is known. However, liver cancer can also occur in healthy individuals for whom there is no known reason.

Risk factors

The following variables raise the chance of developing primary liver cancer:

- **Chronic infection with HBV or HCV:** Liver cancer risk is increased by persistent infection with either the hepatitis B virus (HBV) or the hepatitis C virus (HCV).

- **Cirrhosis:** The formation of scar tissue in your liver as a result of this gradual and irreversible disorder raises your risk of acquiring liver cancer.

- **Certain inherited liver diseases:** Hemochromatosis and Wilson's disease are two liver conditions that can raise the risk of liver cancer.

- **Diabetes:** Compared to people without diabetes, those who have this blood sugar condition are more likely to develop liver cancer.
- **Nonalcoholic fatty liver disease:** Liver cancer risk is increased by a buildup of fat in the liver.
- **Exposure to aflatoxins:** Poisons known as aflatoxins are created when molds develop on improperly stored crops. Aflatoxin contamination can occur in crops like grains and nuts, and the tainted crops can then find their way into meals.
- **Excessive alcohol consumption:** Over many years, drinking more alcohol than is moderately recommended can cause irreversible liver damage and raise your risk of developing liver cancer.

Cirrhosis

Severe liver scarring is known as cirrhosis. Numerous types of liver diseases and disorders, including hepatitis and prolonged alcoholism, can contribute to this dangerous situation.

Your liver attempts to heal itself every time it sustains damage, whether from excessive alcohol use or another factor like an infection. Scar tissue occurs throughout this procedure. An increasing amount of scar tissue grows as cirrhosis worsens, which complicates the liver's ability to function. Advanced cirrhosis can be fatal.

In most cases, cirrhosis-related liver damage is irreversible. However, additional harm can be prevented if liver cirrhosis is identified early and the underlying cause is addressed. Rarely, it might be the opposite.

Symptoms

Many times, cirrhosis is asymptomatic until significant liver damage occurs. When symptoms do appear, they could consist of:

- Fatigue
- easily bruised or bleeding
- appetite decline

- emesis
- Edema is the term for swelling in the ankles, foot, or legs.
- Loss of weight
- Skin irritation
- Jaundice is a yellow coloring of the skin and eyes.
- Ascites, or buildup of fluid in the abdomen
- Skin-surface spider-like blood vessels
- Redness on the hands' palms
- nails that are pale, particularly on the thumb and index finger
- Finger clubbing: a condition where the tips expand out and become more rounded than normal
- Period loss or absence in women is unrelated to menopause
- Gynecomastia, or male breast augmentation, testicular shrinking, or loss of sex desire
- fuzziness, fatigue, or slurred speech.

When to see a doctor

If you experience any of the aforementioned symptoms, schedule a visit with your physician.

Causes

Numerous illnesses and ailments have the potential to harm the liver and cause cirrhosis. Among the reasons are a few of them being:

- chronic misuse of alcohol.
- persistent viral hepatitis (B, C, and D).
- Fat builds up in the liver in a condition known as nonalcoholic fatty liver disease.
- A disorder called hemochromatosis leads to an accumulation of iron in the body.
- An illness of the liver brought on by the immune system is called autoimmune hepatitis.
- bile duct destruction brought on by primary biliary cholangitis.
- biliary duct hardening and scarring brought on by primary sclerosing cholangitis.
- Wilson's illness is a disorder where the liver collects copper.
- fibrosis cystic.

- deficit of alpha-1 antitrypsin.
- Biliary atresia, or poorly developed bile ducts, is a medical disorder.
- genetic diseases related to the metabolism of sugar, such as glycogen storage disease and galactosemia.
- Gastrointestinal genetic condition Alagille syndrome.
- Infection, such as brucellosis or syphilis.
- Medications, including isoniazid or methotrexate.

Risk factors

- **Drinking too much alcohol:** Drinking too much alcohol increases the risk of developing cirrhosis.
- **Being overweight:** Obesity raises the chances of nonalcoholic fatty liver disease and nonalcoholic steatohepatitis, two disorders that can cause cirrhosis.
- **Having viral hepatitis:** Although cirrhosis is one of the main causes of liver disease worldwide, not everyone with chronic hepatitis will go on to develop it.

Complications

Cirrhosis complications can include:

- **High blood pressure in the veins that supply the liver:** Portal hypertension is the name given to this illness. The normal flow of blood through the liver is slowed by cirrhosis. The vein that supplies blood to the liver becomes more pressurized as a result.

- **Swelling in the legs and abdomen:** Ascites, or an accumulation of fluid in the abdomen, and edema, or swelling in the legs, are two possible outcomes of elevated portal vein pressure. When the liver is unable to produce enough albumin or other blood proteins, edema and ascites may also occur.

- **Enlargement of the spleen:** White blood cells and platelets may become trapped in the spleen as a result of portal hypertension. Splenomegaly is the term for the swelling of the spleen caused by this. The initial indication of cirrhosis may be a decrease in white blood cells and platelets in the blood.

- **Bleeding:** Blood can be diverted into smaller veins as a result of portal hypertension. These tiny veins may break due to the increased pressure, resulting in significant bleeding. Varices, or swollen veins, can also result from portal hypertension and occur in the stomach or esophagus. Additionally, these varices may cause potentially fatal hemorrhage. Another reason that may lead to ongoing bleeding is the liver's inability to produce adequate clotting factors.

- **Infections:** It may be difficult for your body to fight infections if you have cirrhosis. Bacterial peritonitis is a dangerous infection that can result from ascites.

- **Malnutrition:** Your body may have a harder time processing nutrients if you have cirrhosis, which could result in weakness and weight loss.

- **Buildup of toxins in the brain:** Toxins cannot be eliminated from the blood as well by a liver damaged by cirrhosis as it can be by a healthy liver. Subsequently, these poisons may accumulate in the brain, leading to cognitive impairment and disorientation. Hepatic encephalopathy is the term for this. Hepatic encephalopathy can eventually lead to a coma or loss of consciousness.

- **Jaundice:** When your sick liver is unable to sufficiently eliminate bilirubin, a blood waste product, from your blood, jaundice develops. Urine turns black and the skin and whites of the eyes turn yellow due to jaundice.

- **Bone disease:** Some cirrhosis patients experience a loss of bone mass and an increased risk of fractures.

- **Increased risk of liver cancer:** Cirrhosis predisposes a significant number of liver cancer patients.

- **Acute-on-chronic cirrhosis:** Some patients eventually have multiple organ failure. It is currently thought by researchers that this is a problem that affects certain cirrhosis patients. They aren't entirely sure what causes it, though.

Autoimmune Hepatitis

When your body's immune system attacks liver cells, it can lead to inflammation of the liver, known as autoimmune hepatitis. Although the precise origin of autoimmune hepatitis is unknown, it seems that over time, environmental and genetic variables interact to develop the illness.

Liver failure may result from untreated autoimmune hepatitis, which can cause cirrhosis, or scarring of the liver. However, immune-suppressive medications are frequently effective in controlling autoimmune hepatitis when the condition is identified and treated early.

If medication is ineffective for treating autoimmune hepatitis or if the liver disease is advanced, a liver transplant may be necessary.

Symptoms

Autoimmune hepatitis symptoms can appear rapidly and vary from person to person. In the early stages of the condition, some persons have few, if any, recognizable issues, while others have signs and symptoms that could include:

- Weary
- discomfort in the abdomen
- Jaundice is the yellowing of the skin and the whites of the eyes.
- An enlarged liver
- Skin blood vessels that are not normal (spider angiomas)
- Rashes on the skin
- joint discomfort
- discontinuation of menstruation

When to see a doctor

Schedule a visit with your physician if you are concerned about any symptoms or indicators.

Causes

When the body's immune system, which normally targets bacteria, viruses, and other pathogens, instead targets the liver, it might result in autoimmune hepatitis. This assault on your liver has the potential to cause severe liver cell destruction as well as persistent inflammation. Although the exact reason of the body's self-destruction remains unknown, scientists believe that exposure to specific viruses or medications along with genes that regulate immune system function may result in autoimmune hepatitis.

Types of autoimmune Hepatitis

Physicians have distinguished between two primary types of autoimmune hepatitis.

- **Type 1 autoimmune hepatitis:** This is the disease's most prevalent form. It is possible at any age. Rheumatoid arthritis, ulcerative colitis, and celiac disease are among the various autoimmune diseases that almost half of those with type 1 autoimmune hepatitis have.

- **Type 2 autoimmune hepatitis:** Type 2 autoimmune hepatitis is more frequent in children and young adults, while it can strike adults as well. This kind of autoimmune hepatitis may coexist with other autoimmune disorders.

Risk factors

The following variables may raise your risk of developing autoimmune hepatitis:

- **Being female:** While autoimmune hepatitis can strike either gender, females are more likely to get it.
- **A history of certain infections:** After contracting the Epstein-Barr virus, herpes simplex, or measles, you may develop autoimmune hepatitis. An infection with hepatitis A, B, or C is also connected to the illness.
- **Heredity:** There is evidence to show that autoimmune hepatitis may run in families.

- **Having an autoimmune disease:** An increased risk of developing autoimmune hepatitis exists in those with pre-existing autoimmune diseases, such as celiac disease, rheumatoid arthritis, or hyperthyroidism (also known as Graves' disease or Hashimoto's thyroiditis).

Complications

If left untreated, autoimmune hepatitis can result in cirrhosis, a persistent scarring of the liver tissue. Cirrhosis complications consist of:

- **Enlarged veins in your esophagus (esophageal varices):** Blood may back up into other blood vessels, primarily the esophageal and stomach blood vessels, when circulation through the portal vein is obstructed. Because the blood arteries have thin walls and are carrying more blood than they should, bleeding is prone to occur. Severe bleeding from these blood vessels in the stomach or esophagus is a potentially fatal situation that needs to be treated right once.

- **Fluid in your abdomen (ascites):** Your abdomen may fill up with a lot of fluid if you have liver illness. Ascites is typically an indication of severe cirrhosis and can be painful as well as cause respiratory difficulties.
- **Liver failure:** This happens when your liver can no longer function normally due to significant damage to the liver cells. Currently, a liver transplant is required.
- **Liver cancer:** Liver cancer is more common in those with cirrhosis.

Hemochromatosis

Your body absorbs too much iron from food if you have hemochromatosis. Your organs, particularly the liver, heart, and pancreas, accumulate excess iron. Life-threatening illnesses like diabetes, heart difficulties, and liver disease can be brought on by an excess of iron.

Hemochromatosis comes in various forms, but the most prevalent kind is inherited due to a genetic alteration. Few individuals with the genes ever have significant issues. Midlife is when symptoms typically manifest.

A typical part of treatment is having blood drawn from your body. This medication decreases iron levels because red blood cells hold a large amount of the body's iron.

Symptoms

Hemochromatosis may never cause symptoms in certain individuals. Early signs and symptoms of other common illnesses frequently coexist.

Among the symptoms could be:

- Joint discomfort
- stomach ache
- Weakness and Fatigue
- Diabetes
- reduction in sex desire
- Ineffectiveness
- heart attack
- Failure of the liver
- Gray or bronze skin tone
- fog in the memory.

Hemochromatosis of the most prevalent kind is inherited. However, the majority of people don't exhibit symptoms until later in life; for women, this usually happens after age 60 and for men, after age 40. After menopause, when they no longer lose iron through menstruation and pregnancy, women are more likely to experience symptoms.

When to see a doctor

If you encounter any hemochromatosis symptoms, consult your physician. Consult your healthcare practitioner about genetic testing if you have hemochromatosis in any members of your immediate family. You can find out if you carry the gene that makes hemochromatosis more likely by having a genetic test.

Causes

Gene mutations are the most common cause of hemochromatosis. This gene regulates how much iron is absorbed by the body through diet. Children inherit the mutated gene from their parents. By far the most prevalent kind of hemochromatosis is this one. Hereditary hemochromatosis is the term for it.

Gene mutations that cause hemochromatosis

The most common cause of hereditary hemochromatosis is a gene called HFE. One HFE gene is inherited from each parent. There are two frequent mutations in the HFE gene: C282Y and H63D. You can find out if you have these mutations in your HFE gene through genetic testing.

- Hemochromatosis can occur if you inherit two mutated genes. The mutated gene can potentially be inherited by your offspring. However, not all individuals who receive two genes experience issues related to hemochromatosis' iron overload.

- Hemochromatosis is not likely to occur if you inherit one mutated gene. On the other hand, you are thought to be a carrier of the mutation [altered gene], which you can then pass on to your progeny. However, unless your children also got another changed gene from the other parent, they would not have the condition.

How hemochromatosis affects your organs

Among the many vital bodily processes iron aids in is blood production. Yet an excess of iron is harmful.

Hepcidin, a hormone released by the liver, regulates the body's usage and absorption of iron. It also regulates the organs' storage of excess iron. Hepcidin's function is compromised in hemochromatosis, leading to the body absorbing more iron than it requires.

The liver, in particular, stores a large amount of this extra iron. The iron that has been accumulated can seriously harm organs over years and even result in organ failure. Long-term conditions including cirrhosis, diabetes, and heart failure can also result from it. Hemochromatosis is a result of gene mutations that affect many people. But not everyone has iron overload to the point where organ and tissue damage results.

There are other types of hemochromatosis besides hereditary hemochromatosis. Additional varieties consist of:

- **Juvenile hemochromatosis:** In young people, this results in the same issues that adult hereditary hemochromatosis brings. However, iron accumulation starts considerably earlier, with symptoms typically manifesting between the ages of 15 and 30. Gene alterations related to hemojuvelin or hepcidin cause this illness.

- **Neonatal hemochromatosis:** In this serious condition, iron accumulates quickly in the growing fetus's liver. It is believed to be an autoimmune illness, meaning the body targets itself.

- **Secondary hemochromatosis:** This type of the illness, which goes by the name "iron overload," is not inherited. Individuals who suffer from specific forms of anemia or liver disease may require repeated transfusions of blood. Excess iron accumulation may result from this.

Risk factors

Hemochromatosis is caused by a number of factors, which include:

- **Family history:** You have an increased risk of hemochromatosis if you have a parent or sibling who has the condition.

- **Having two copies of an altered HFE gene:** The biggest cause of hereditary hemochromatosis is this.

- **Your sex:** Hemochromatosis symptoms are more likely to appear in men than in women early in life. Women tend to keep less iron than males do because they lose it during pregnancy and menstruation. For women, the risk increases following menopause or a hysterectomy.

- **Ethnicity:** Hereditary hemochromatosis is more common in people of Northern European heritage than in people of other ethnic backgrounds. Asian, Hispanic, and

Black individuals are less likely to have hemochromatosis.

Complications

Hemochromatosis can result in several consequences if left untreated. Particularly affected by these issues are your joints and organs, such as the liver, pancreas, and heart, which are known to accumulate extra iron. Among the complications are:

- **Liver problems:** A persistent scarring of the liver called cirrhosis is one of the issues that can arise. Liver cancer and other potentially fatal consequences are among the risks associated with cirrhosis.

- **Diabetes:** Diabetes may result from pancreatic damage.

- **Heart problems:** The ability of your heart to pump enough blood to meet your body's needs is impacted by having too much iron in it. We refer to this as congestive heart failure. Hemochromatosis can also result in arrhythmias, which are irregular cardiac beats.

- **Reproductive problems:** Men who have too much iron may experience erectile dysfunction and a decrease in sex desire. In women, it may result in the cessation of the menstrual cycle.
- **Skin color changes:** Your skin may appear gray or bronze due to iron deposits in skin cells.

Wilson's Disease

Wilson's illness is an uncommon hereditary disorder that results in an accumulation of copper in multiple organs, including the brain, eyes, and liver. Between the ages of 5 and 35, Wilson's illness is diagnosed in the majority of cases. However, both young and old might be impacted.

Building strong bones, collagen, nerves, and the skin pigment melanin all depend on copper. Copper is typically ingested through food. Any excess copper is eliminated via the bile that your liver generates.

However, copper is not adequately eliminated in those who have Wilson's disease; instead, it accumulates. If left untreated, it occasionally poses a life-threatening risk. Wilson's disease is treatable when detected early, and many affected individuals lead normal lives.

Symptoms

Wilson's illness is present from birth, but symptoms don't show up until the liver, brain, eyes, or another organ starts to accumulate copper. The portions of your body that are affected by the disease determine the symptoms.

Among these symptoms are the following:

- weariness and appetite decline.
- Jaundice is the term for a yellowing of the skin and the whites of the eyes.
- Kayser-Fleischer rings are the golden-brown or copper-colored bands that encircle the eye's irises.
- accumulation of fluid in the stomach or legs.
- difficulties swallowing, speaking, or moving physically coordinated.
- Depression, shifts in mood, and modifications in personality.

- experiencing difficulty going to sleep and remaining asleep.
- Involuntary motions or rigidity in muscles.

When to see a doctor

If you have symptoms that concern you, schedule a visit with your physician or another primary care provider. This is especially important if you have a family member with Wilson's disease.

Causes

Wilson's disease results from a mutated gene that is inherited from both parents. You will be a carrier but not an actual patient if you have only one mutated gene. This implies that your offspring may inherit the impacted gene.

Risk factors

Wilson's illness may be more common in you if it affects your parents or siblings. To determine whether you have Wilson's disease, ask your doctor if genetic testing is necessary. Early diagnosis of the illness significantly improves the prognosis for recovery.

Complications

Wilson's disease can occasionally be fatal if left untreated. Significant side effects consist of:

- **Scarring of the liver, also known as cirrhosis:** Scar tissue develops in the liver when hepatic cells attempt to repair damage brought on by elevated copper levels. The liver has a tougher time functioning as a result.

- **Liver failure:** This condition, sometimes referred to as decompensated Wilson's disease or acute liver failure, can strike unexpectedly. It may also develop gradually over several years. One course of treatment could be a liver transplant.

- **Lasting nervous system issues:** With Wilson's disease treatment, tremors, involuntary muscular movements, clumsy walking, and difficulty speaking normally improve. However, even after receiving treatment, some patients continue to have neurological system issues.

- **Kidney problems:** Kidney damage from Wilson's disease can result in problems including kidney stones and an abnormally high amount of amino acids eliminated in the urine.

- **Mental health issues:** These could include psychosis, bipolar illness, depression, irritability, or changes in personality.
- **Blood problems:** Hemolysis, the term for the breakdown of red blood cells, is one of these. This results in jaundice and anemia.

Primary Biliary Cholangitis

An autoimmune condition known as primary biliary cholangitis causes inflammation and gradual bile duct destruction. It was formerly known as primary cirrhosis of the liver.

The liver produces a fluid called bile. It facilitates vitamin absorption and digestion. In addition, it aids in the body's absorption of lipids and the removal of toxins, cholesterol, and worn-out red blood cells. Chronic inflammation of the liver can cause cholangitis, or inflammation and damage to the bile ducts. This occasionally results in cirrhosis, a permanent scarring of the liver tissue. Liver failure may possibly eventually result from it. Primary biliary cholangitis primarily affects women, though it can affect both sexes. Since it's classified as an autoimmune illness, your body's immune system is unintentionally targeting healthy tissue and cells. Scientists believe the illness is brought on by a confluence of environmental and genetic variables. Usually, it progresses slowly. Primary biliary cholangitis currently has no known cure, however medications may lessen liver damage, particularly if treatment starts early.

Symptoms

When primary biliary cholangitis is diagnosed, about half of the patients do not exhibit any symptoms. When blood tests are performed for other purposes, including routine testing, the disease may be identified. Over the following five to twenty years, symptoms gradually appear. Those with symptoms at diagnosis usually don't fare as well.

Exhaustion and irritated skin are frequent initial signs.

Subsequent indications and symptoms could be:

- Jaundice is the term for a yellowing of the skin and eyes.
- lips and eyes dry.
- abdominal pain in the upper right corner.
- Splenomegaly is the term for splenic swelling.
- joint, muscle, or bone aches.
- ankles and feet swelling.
- Ascites is the accumulation of fluid in the abdomen as a result of liver failure.
- Fatty deposits on the skin near the eyes, on the eyelids, or in the creases of the elbows, knees, palms, or soles are referred to as xanthomas.
- Hyperpigmentation is the term for skin darkening unrelated to sun exposure.
- Osteoporosis is a condition that causes weak, fragile bones that can break.
- elevated cholesterol.

- Steatorrhea is a type of diarrhea that might include oily stools.
- Hypothyroidism, the underactive thyroid
- Reduced weight.

Causes

The etiology of primary biliary cholangitis is unknown. According to many specialists, it's an autoimmune disease where the body attacks its own cells. Researchers think that both hereditary and environmental factors may cause this autoimmune reaction.

Primary biliary cholangitis is characterized by inflammation of the liver that develops from the accumulation of T cells, commonly referred to as T lymphocytes, a subset of white blood cells. These immune cells typically identify and aid in the defense against bacteria, viruses, and other pathogens. However, they unintentionally kill the healthy cells lining the liver's tiny bile channels when treating primary biliary cholangitis.

The smallest ducts become inflamed, which then spreads and affects more liver cells. When the cells die, scar tissue, sometimes referred to as fibrosis, grows in their stead and can eventually cause cirrhosis. The scarring of liver tissue caused by cirrhosis impairs the liver's ability to function normally.

Risk factors

Your chance of developing primary biliary cholangitis may be raised by the following factors:

- **Sex:** It is mostly women that suffer from primary biliary cholangitis.

- **Age:** It most commonly affects those between the ages of 30 and 60.

- **Genetics:** If you have a family member who currently has the illness, your chances of getting it are higher.

- **Geography:** Although illness can affect persons of many races and ethnicities, primary biliary cholangitis is most common in those of northern European ancestry.

Researchers believe that primary biliary cholangitis is caused by a combination of hereditary and environmental factors. These outside elements could consist of:

- infections in the urinary tract, for example.

- smoking tobacco, particularly for extended periods of time.

- exposure to hazardous substances, as in several occupational settings.

Complications

Primary biliary cholangitis can lead to major health issues when liver damage increases, such as:

- **Liver scarring, called cirrhosis:** Liver failure may result from cirrhosis, which impairs the liver's function. It refers to primary biliary cholangitis in its advanced stages. The prognosis for patients with cirrhosis and primary biliary cholangitis is not good. They are also more likely to experience other issues.

- **Increased pressure in the portal vein, called portal hypertension:** The portal vein is a sizable blood channel that allows blood from your pancreas, spleen, and intestines to reach your liver. Blood backs up in your liver when cirrhosis-related scar tissue obstructs normal blood flow through it. The vein's internal pressure rises as a result. Additionally, medicines and other poisons aren't adequately filtered out of your bloodstream because your liver isn't able to process blood flow correctly.

- **Enlarged veins, called varices:** Blood may back up into other veins when the portal vein's blood flow is impeded or obstructed. Usually, it backs up into the esophageal and stomach cavities. Delicate veins may bleed and burst from increased strain. A potentially fatal situation is upper stomach or esophageal bleeding. It needs medical attention right away.

- **Enlarged spleen, called splenomegaly:** It is possible for your spleen to swell with platelets and white blood cells. This occurs as a result of your body's inability to properly filter poisons out of your bloodstream.

- **Gallstones and bile duct stones:** Bile may solidify into stones in the bile ducts if it is unable to pass through them. These stones have the potential to infect and hurt.

- **Liver cancer:** Your risk of liver cancer rises if you have liver scarring. You will require routine cancer screenings if you have liver scarring.

- **Weak bones, called osteoporosis:** Individuals suffering from primary biliary cholangitis are more susceptible to weak, brittle bones that might break more readily.

- **Vitamin deficiencies:** Your digestive system's capacity to absorb lipids and the fat-soluble vitamins A, D, E, and K is impacted when there is insufficient bile. Because of this, low levels of these vitamins may be present in certain patients with advanced primary biliary cholangitis. Low levels can cause bleeding abnormalities and night blindness, among other health issues.

- **High cholesterol:** People with primary biliary cholangitis can have elevated cholesterol in as much as 80% of cases.

- **Decreased mental function, called hepatic encephalopathy:** Personality changes have been reported in some patients with severe primary biliary cholangitis and cirrhosis. They might also struggle with focus and remembering.

- **Increased risk of other disease:** Thyroid, skin, and joint diseases are among the conditions that are linked to primary biliary cholangitis. Additionally, it may be connected to Sjogren's syndrome, a condition characterized by dry lips and eyes.

Primary sclerosing cholangitis

The illness known as primary sclerosing cholangitis affects the bile ducts. The digesting liquid bile is transported from your liver to your small intestine by bile ducts. The bile ducts become scarred as a result of inflammation in primary sclerosing cholangitis. These scars restrict and harden the ducts, which over time seriously damages the liver. Most patients with primary sclerosing cholangitis also have Crohn's disease or ulcerative colitis, two conditions that cause inflammation of the intestines.

Primary sclerosing cholangitis typically advances slowly in its victims. Liver failure, recurrent infections, and bile duct or liver cancers are possible outcomes. Advanced primary sclerosing cholangitis currently has no known treatment other than a liver transplant; nevertheless, a tiny percentage of patients may have recurrence of the illness in their new liver.

Monitoring liver function, treating symptoms, and, where feasible, performing treatments that temporarily unblock blocked bile ducts are the main goals of care for primary sclerosing cholangitis.

Symptoms

When liver abnormalities are seen on a routine blood test or an X-ray obtained for an unrelated ailment, primary sclerosing cholangitis is frequently detected before symptoms manifest.

Typical early warning signs and symptoms are:

- Itching
- Fatigue
- Abdominal pain
- Yellow eyes and skin (jaundice)

Many individuals with primary sclerosing cholangitis who are diagnosed before they exhibit symptoms go years without experiencing any symptoms at all. However, no one can accurately forecast how fast or slowly their particular condition will proceed.

The following are indications and symptoms that could develop as the illness worsens:

- Sweating at night Fever Chills
- enlarged liver
- enlarged spleen
- Loss of weight

When to see a doctor

If you have intense, inexplicable itching across a large portion of your body that won't go away no matter how often you scratch, schedule a visit with your doctor. See your doctor if you experience constant fatigue that does not go away.

It is especially crucial to consult your physician about unexplained exhaustion and itching if you suffer from Crohn's disease or ulcerative colitis, two conditions that fall under the category of inflammatory bowel disease. Most patients with primary sclerosing cholangitis also suffer from one of these conditions.

Causes

The major etiology of sclerosing cholangitis is unknown. In those who are genetically susceptible to the condition, the disease may be brought on by the immune system's response to an infection or toxin.

An extensive percentage of patients with primary sclerosing cholangitis also have inflammatory bowel disease, which is a general phrase that encompasses Crohn's disease and ulcerative colitis.

However, inflammatory bowel disease and primary sclerosing cholangitis don't always manifest themselves together. Primary sclerosing cholangitis can sometimes exist for years prior to the onset of inflammatory bowel disease. Due to the increased risk of colon cancer, it is crucial to search for inflammatory bowel disease if primary sclerosing cholangitis is found.

It happens less frequently for patients receiving treatment for inflammatory bowel disease to also develop primary sclerosing cholangitis. Moreover, inflammatory bowel disease rarely develops in patients with primary sclerosing cholangitis until after a liver transplant.

Risk factors

Factors that may increase the risk of primary sclerosing cholangitis include:

- **Age:** Although primary sclerosing cholangitis can strike at any age, the 30s and 40s are the most common ages at which it is diagnosed.
- **Sex:** There is a higher incidence of primary sclerosing cholangitis in men.

- **Inflammatory bowel disease:** Inflammatory bowel illness coexists with primary sclerosing cholangitis in a significant number of cases.
- **Geographical location:** Individuals having ancestry from Northern Europe are more susceptible to primary sclerosing cholangitis.

Complications

Primary sclerosing cholangitis complications can include:

- **Liver disease and failure:** Chronic inflammation of your liver's bile ducts can cause liver cell death, tissue scarring (cirrhosis), and ultimately loss of liver function.
- **Repeated infections:** You may have recurrent bile duct infections if scarring in the bile ducts reduces or completely blocks the flow of bile from the liver. After a surgical surgery to remove a stone that was obstructing your bile duct or to extend a

severely scarred bile duct, you are especially vulnerable to infection.

Portal hypertension: The main vein that carries blood from your digestive tract to your liver is called the portal vein. In this vein, elevated blood pressure is referred to as portal hypertension.

Ascites, or the leakage of liver fluid into the abdominal cavity, can be caused by portal hypertension. Additionally, it may cause varices, or enlarged veins, in other veins by redirecting blood from the portal vein to those other veins. Varices are fragile veins that bleed readily, which poses a serious risk to life.

- **Thinning bones:** It is possible for people with primary sclerosing cholangitis to have osteoporosis, or thinning bones. Every few years, your doctor could advise a bone density test to check for osteoporosis. To assist prevent bone loss, doctors may prescribe calcium and vitamin D supplements.

- **Bile duct cancer:** You run a higher chance of developing gallbladder or bile duct cancer if you have primary sclerosing cholangitis.

- **Colon cancer:** Colon cancer risk is higher in those with primary sclerosing cholangitis linked to inflammatory bowel disease. Even if you have no symptoms, your doctor may advise testing for inflammatory bowel disease if you have been diagnosed with primary sclerosing cholangitis because having both conditions increases your chance of colon cancer.

Non-Alcoholic fatty liver disease (NAFLD)

People who drink little to no alcohol are susceptible to a liver condition known as nonalcoholic fatty liver disease, or NAFLD for short. In NAFLD, the liver accumulates excessive fat. Obese or overweight folks are the ones who experience it most frequently.

Globally, NAFLD is growing increasingly prevalent as the rate of obesity rises, particularly in Western and Middle Eastern countries. It is the most prevalent type of chronic liver disease, impacting around 25% of people worldwide. Approximately 100 million Americans suffer with NAFLD.

Nonalcoholic steatohepatitis, or NASH, is a condition that some people with NAFLD may develop. Because of the fat deposits in the liver, NASH is a severe type of fatty liver disease that damages and swells the liver. As NASH worsens, it may cause severe liver damage known as cirrhosis and possibly even liver cancer. The harm induced by excessive alcohol use is similar to this harm.

Currently, there is a movement to rename the condition as metabolic dysfunction-associated steatotic liver disease (MASLD) instead of nonalcoholic fatty liver disease. Additionally, experts suggest renaming the condition metabolic dysfunction-associated steatohepatitis (MASH) instead of nonalcoholic steatohepatitis.

Symptoms NAFLD frequently exhibits none at all. When it does, these could consist of:

- Weariness.

- Malaise, or not feeling well.
- discomfort or pain in the upper right abdomen.

The following are potential signs of cirrhosis, or extensive scarring, and NASH:

- Skin irritation
- Also known as ascites, abdominal swelling
- breathing difficulty Leg swelling
- Spider-like blood veins that are barely visible through the skin
- enlarged spleen
- crimson hands
- Jaundice is the yellowing of the skin and eyes.

When to see a doctor

If you are concerned about any persistent symptoms, schedule a visit with a member of your healthcare team.

causes

The specific reason why fat accumulates in certain livers but not in others is unknown to experts. Additionally, they are not entirely sure why some fatty livers develop NASH.

The following are connected to both NAFLD and NASH:

- Obesity or being overweight
- Genetics
- Insulin resistance, often known as hyperglycemia or elevated blood sugar, is the result of your cells' inability to absorb sugar in response to the insulin hormone. Type 2 diabetes
- elevated blood fat levels, particularly in triglycerides.

The accumulation of these medical conditions could lead to a fatty liver. Nonetheless, some persons can still develop NAFLD even in the absence of risk factors.

Risk factors

The following conditions and illnesses can raise your risk of NAFLD:

- obesity or fatty liver disease in the family history
- Insufficient production of growth hormones in the body results in growth hormone deficit.

- elevated cholesterol.
- elevated blood triglyceride levels.
- resistance to insulin.
- syndrome of metabolism.
- obesity, particularly when the bulk of the fat is around the waist.
- syndrome of polycystic ovary.
- apnea obstructive sleep.
- diabetes type 2.
- Hypothyroidism, or underactive thyroid,
- hypopituitarism, or underactivity of the pituitary gland.

These groups are more prone to have NASH:

- Individuals over the age of fifty
- Individuals who possess specific genetic risk factors
- Obese Individuals
- Individuals who have high blood sugar or diabetes
- those who exhibit high blood pressure, high triglycerides, and a big waist size—symptoms of metabolic syndrome.

NAFLD and NASH are difficult to distinguish from one another without a clinical assessment and testing.

Complications

cirrhosis, or severe liver scarring, is the primary NAFLD and NASH consequence. Liver injury, such as that brought on by NASH inflammation, results in cirrhosis. The liver produces regions of scarring, also known as fibrosis, in an attempt to reduce inflammation. As the inflammation persists, the fibrosis expands and consumes more liver tissue.

If the scarring is not stopped, cirrhosis may result in:

- Ascites is an accumulation of fluid in the stomach region.
- varices, or swollen veins in the esophagus, that have the potential to burst and hemorrhage.
- Hepatic encephalopathy is another term for confusion, drowsiness, and slurred speech.

- Hypersplenism, or an overactive spleen, can result in insufficient blood platelets.

- carcinoma of the liver.

- end-stage liver failure: this indicates that the liver is no longer functional.

Experts estimate that 1.5% to 6.5% of adults in the United States have NASH, and roughly 24% have NAFLD.

Prevention of Alcoholic Hepatitis

Your chance of developing alcoholic hepatitis may be lower if you:

- If you use alcohol at all, do it in moderation. One drink per day for women and two drinks per day for males is considered moderate drinking for healthy individuals. Eliminating alcohol completely is the only surefire method to prevent alcoholic hepatitis.

- Defend against contracting hepatitis C. A virus causes the liver illness known as hepatitis C. If left untreated, it might develop into cirrhosis. Drinking alcohol increases your risk of developing cirrhosis if you have hepatitis C.

- Make sure before combining drink and medication. Find out from your healthcare provider whether it's okay to have alcohol while taking your recommended medications. Examine the warning labels on over-the-counter medications. When using medications that advise against consuming alcohol while taking them, do not consume alcohol. This contains analgesics like acetaminophen (found in Tylenol and other brands).

Prevention of Liver Cancer

Reduce your risk of cirrhosis

Liver cancer risk is increased by cirrhosis, which causes scarring of the liver. You can lower the chance of developing cirrhosis if you:

- If you use alcohol at all, do it in moderation. If you decide to consume alcohol, keep your intake to a minimum. This translates to women having no more than one drink each day. This translates to guys having no more than two drinks each day.

- Sustain a healthy weight. If you are currently at a healthy weight, make an effort to stay there by eating well and doing exercise most days of the week. Lower your daily calorie intake and up your workout regimen if you need to shed some weight. Aim for weekly weight loss of one or two pounds (0.5 to 1 kg).

- Obtain a hepatitis B vaccination: Getting vaccinated against hepatitis B can lower your risk of contracting the disease. Nearly everyone can receive the vaccination, including young children, elderly people, and people with weakened immune systems.

- Take precautions against contracting hepatitis C: Hepatitis C has no known vaccination, but you can lower your chance of contracting the illness.

- Any sexual partner's health status should be known. Unless you are positive that your partner is free of HBV, HCV, or any other sexually transmitted virus, avoid having unprotected intercourse. Use a condom each and every time you engage in sexual activity with someone you don't know well.

- Avoid using intravenous (IV) medications, but if you must, make sure the needle is clean. Reducing your risk of HIV by abstaining from illicit drug injection. If that's not an option for you, however, make sure that any needle you use is sterile and dispose of it properly. An infection with hepatitis C is frequently caused by tainted medication accessories. Use the needle-exchange services in your area, and think about getting drug treatment.

- When getting a tattoo or getting pierced, look for clean, safe shops. Unsterilized needles have the potential to transmit the hepatitis C virus. Examine local stores for piercings and tattoos and inquire with staff about their safety procedures before having one. You can tell If a store isn't the proper place for you if the staff doesn't want to talk to you or doesn't think your queries are important.

- Seek medical attention if you have hepatitis B or C. Both hepatitis B and hepatitis C illnesses have treatments available. Treatment can lower the risk of liver cancer, according to research.

Consult your physician about screening for liver cancer. It is not usually advised to screen for liver cancer in the general population as there is no evidence that doing so lowers the chance of dying from the disease. Individuals who have any of the following conditions that raise their risk of liver cancer should think about getting screened:

- Hepatitis B infection
- Hepatitis C infection
- Liver cirrhosis

Examine the benefits and drawbacks of screening with your physician. Based on your risk, you can determine together if screening is appropriate for you. Every six months, a blood test and an abdominal ultrasound examination are usually part of the screening process.

Prevention of Cirrhosis

Consider these measures to take better care of your liver and reduce your chance of cirrhosis:

- Avoid alcohol consumption if you have cirrhosis. Alcohol use is not advised if you have liver illness.

- Consume a balanced diet. Make fruit and vegetable-rich diet choices. Make sure to use lean protein sources and nutritious carbohydrates. Reduce the quantity of fried and fatty foods you consume.

- Sustain a healthy weight. Overindulgence in fat might harm your liver. If you are obese or overweight, discuss a weight-loss plan with your healthcare physician.

Cut down on your hepatitis risk. Hepatitis B and C can be contracted through unprotected intercourse and sharing of needles. Find out from your doctor about hepatitis immunizations.

Consult your healthcare professional about strategies to lower your risk of liver cirrhosis if you're worried about it.

Prevention of NAFLD

To reduce your risk of NAFLD:

- Consume a balanced diet. Consume a diet high in fruits, vegetables, whole grains, and healthy fats to maintain good health.

- Cut back on simple sweets, alcohol, and portion sizes. Steer clear of sugary beverages including sweet tea, soda, sports drinks, and juices. Alcohol use should be restricted or avoided as it can harm your liver.

- Maintain a healthy weight. Collaborate with your medical team to progressively reduce your weight if you are fat or overweight. Maintain a healthy weight by eating a balanced diet and doing regular exercise.

- Work out. Make the most of your daily activities. If you haven't been exercising consistently, get the go-ahead from your medical team beforehand.

You probably don't give it much thought, yet your liver plays a vital role in the digestive system of your body. It filters everything you eat, drink, and even medications. It needs proper care in order for it to remain healthy and perform as intended.

If you don't take proper care of it, you could quickly ruin this organ, and once you do, it's gone.

Located beneath your lower ribs on the right side, your liver is roughly the size of a football. It must do a number of crucial tasks. It helps purify your blood by eliminating toxic substances that are produced by your body. It produces bile, a fluid that aids in the breakdown of fat in diet. Additionally, it stores glucose, a type of sugar that, when needed, provides a rapid energy boost.

Maintaining the health of your liver is not difficult. Maintaining a healthy lifestyle is crucial. Avoiding harmful things is considerably more important for liver health than consuming foods or beverages that are especially beneficial to the liver.

These are some tips to maintain the health of your liver:

- **Don't drink a lot of alcohol:** It can harm liver cells and cause inflammation or scarring that develops into cirrhosis, a potentially fatal condition. According to US government guidelines, women should have one drink per day and males should have no more than two.

- **Eat a healthy diet and get regular exercise:** Your liver will be appreciative. You'll avoid nonalcoholic fatty liver disease

(NAFLD), which is a condition that can develop to cirrhosis, by maintaining a healthy weight.

Watch out for certain medicines: Liver issues may occasionally arise as a side effect of certain cholesterol medications. Acetaminophen, the painkiller found in Tylenol, might damage your liver if you consume too much of it.

It's possible that you're taking more acetaminophen than you know. It is present in hundreds of medications, including prescription pain relievers and cold remedies.

When taking some medications, drinking alcohol can cause liver damage. And some become dangerous when mixed with other medications. The safest way to take your medications should be discussed with your doctor or pharmacist.

- **Learn how to prevent viral hepatitis:** It's a dangerous condition that damages your liver. There are various kinds. Eating or drinking water contaminated with the hepatitis A virus can expose you to the virus. If you are going to a region of the world where there are epidemics, you can receive a vaccination. Hepatitis B and C can be transmitted by bodily fluids such as blood. Share not things like needles, toothbrushes, or razors to reduce your risk. Restrict the amount of sexual partners you have, and use latex condoms at all times. Hepatitis B has a vaccine, but there is currently none for hepatitis C.

Obtain a viral hepatitis test. It is generally asymptomatic, so you may have it for years without realizing it. See your doctor to determine whether you require a blood test if you believe you have come into contact with the virus.

The CDC advises anyone born between 1945 and 1965 to have a hepatitis C test. The condition is more common in the baby boomer age.

- **Don't touch or breathe in toxins:** Certain aerosol items, pesticides, and cleaning supplies contain compounds that are harmful to the liver. Steer clear of direct interaction with them. Don't smoke because the additives in cigarettes might harm your liver as well.

  Use caution when consuming herbs and dietary supplements. There are some that can damage your liver: A handful that have been problematic include ephedra, kava, cascara, chaparral, and comfrey.

  There have been pills and botanicals on the market recently that claim to heal the liver. Don't believe their assertions. No credible research has ever shown that any of these supports liver health. Some might even be harmful.

Drink coffee: It can reduce your risk of developing liver disease, according to research. Nobody is sure why this is the case, but as more study is done, it's important to monitor.

Maintain a healthy lifestyle and pay special attention to medications to keep your liver in good condition. Although the liver has its limitations, it may be a remarkably forgiving organ.

The End